Law of Attr

Weight

Change Your Relationship with Food, Stop Torturing Yourself with "Dieting" and Transform Your Body with LOA!

By Elena G.Rivers

Disclaimer Notice:

Please note the information contained in this document is for educational and entertainment purposes only. Every attempt has been made to provide accurate, up to date and completely reliable information. No warranties of any kind are expressed or implied.

Readers acknowledge that the author is not engaging in the rendering of legal, financial, medical or professional advice. By reading this document, the reader agrees that under no circumstances are we responsible for any losses, direct or indirect, which are incurred as a result of the use of information contained within this document, including, but not limited to, errors, omissions, or inaccuracies.

Weight Loss Guidance from the Universe:
How to Transform Your Body (and mind) with the Law of Attraction

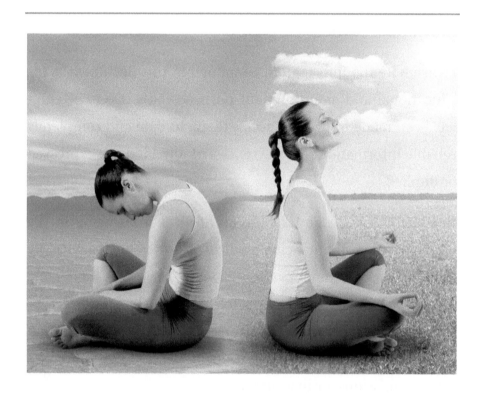

Contents

Introduction

Why write a book on weight loss using the Law of Attraction? Why pick such an esoteric subject? After all, there are plenty of books that are available on the Law of Attraction and even more books on weight loss. At first, I thought it was a crazy idea. However, after giving it more thought, I realized what a genius idea it was.

I have written numerous guides on the Law of Attraction. However, I always felt frustrated that I was unable to fully express my thoughts about it. I was unable to express my feelings about it adequately because the Law of Attraction operates beyond the level of thought. Rather, a thought is an expression of the Law of Attraction, and the Law of Attraction is a manifestation of universal consciousness or energy.

Linking weight loss to the Law of Attraction makes it an ideal vehicle to explain the Law of Attraction in a way that most people can relate to. Weight loss is a perfect metaphor for describing how societal indoctrination has caused us to lose our connection with ourselves, other people, and the natural world. We have established our sense of self on our physical body and our beliefs, which leads us to engage in a war with ourselves to conform to societal standards.

Given all that I have written so far, let me say to you that this weight loss book will be unlike any weight loss book you have ever read. You will not find any diet plans or nutritional recommendations, nor will you find any physical exercises prescribed. There is a deluge of content that covers these things, which is why weight loss is a never-ending struggle for most people.

The typical weight loss book does not address the cause. Rather, it regards the symptoms of that cause. What is this cause I speak of? We are multi-dimensional beings who live simultaneously as non-physical beings and a mind with a physical body. It is our sense of separation from our most fundamental nature, which is consciousness, which has left us feeling that we are missing something from our lives, that somehow we are flawed. We believe this because we compare ourselves to others who are also experiencing a sense of separation from their highest nature.

We are like a king who is experiencing amnesia. Because he has forgotten that he comes from royalty, he spends his days believing that he is a peasant. This book was written as a reminder to you, the reader, that you can remember your higher truth and transform your life by transforming your mind and body.

Lastly, I mentioned that this book uses weight loss as a vehicle for the purpose of creating a deeper understanding of the Law of Attraction. Because of this, this book is relevant to any struggle that you may be experiencing. You can replace "weight loss" with the challenge that you are facing, be it smoking, anger, shyness, low self-esteem, or any other problem that you can think of. After all, they are all symptoms, but there is only one cause.

The first part of this book will provide information regarding the Law of Attraction, the nature of consciousness, and identity.

The second part of this book will discuss how weight loss relates to the Law of Attraction and practical steps that you can take to apply it to weight loss. One final note, the topic of this book involves using terms to explain things that are beyond our ability to conceive with the mind.

Because of this, do not take any terms in this book literally. Rather, trust your feelings as you read the book and determine what is right for you.

Throughout this book, I have tried to use different terms to describe that which is indescribable. Do not try do differentiate between consciousness, the universe, or the higher self, as they are all intended to refer to the same thing.

Before we get into it...I want to offer you a free gift and free access to my VIP LOA Newsletter. See you on the next page☺

A Special Offer from Elena to Help You Manifest Faster.

The best way to get in touch with me is by joining my free email newsletter.

You can easily do it in a few seconds by visiting our private website at:

www.Loaforsuccess.com/newsletter

The best part?

When you sign up, you will instantly receive a free copy of an exclusive LOA Workbook that will help you raise your vibration in 5 days or less:

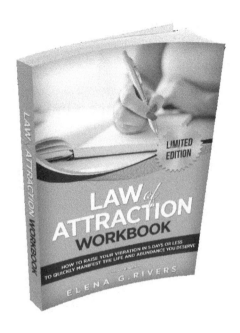

You will also be the first one to learn about my new releases, bonuses and other valuable resources to help you on your journey.

Sign up now and I'll "see you" in the first email.

Love,

Elena

Recovering from the Amnesia

"If you change the way you look at things, the things you look at change."

-Wayne Dyer

I would like to start this chapter with a simple, yet profound exercise. Think of this exercise as setting the mood, just as you would if you were preparing a romantic dinner for a special date. In this case, that date is an aspect of you that you have most likely forgotten about. Do the following:

1. Find a comfortable place to sit and close your eyes.
2. I want you to just relax by focusing on your breath. Breathe normally and make it the focus of your attention.
3. As you focus on your breath, do not make any effort to change anything. Do not hold any expectations or have any anticipations of what may happen during the course of this exercise. Do not get caught up with your thinking. If a thought appears, just return your focus to your breath.

4. Do not hold on to any thoughts of the past. Do not hold on to any thoughts that you may have about yourself, other people, or your situation.

5. Do not entertain any thoughts of your desires, goals, or responsibilities.

6. Do not give any of your attention to thoughts of doing this exercise correctly, or your doubts, or fears.

7. Though thoughts, feelings, and sensations will present themselves to you. Do not get involved with them. Offer them your complete acceptance and continue to focus on your breath.

Continue with this exercise in this manner until you experience a sense of stillness and calm. When experiencing that stillness and quiet, take the time to enjoy it. If the silence or calmness seems to fade away, do not worry about it. Do not try to control it. Accept whatever you are experiencing; the stillness and calm will return. That statement is not entirely correct. The stillness and peace never leave you; they are always there. What appears to be the stillness fading away is your mind focusing on something else. What is this stillness? The stillness that you experience is your connecting with your higher truth. Your essential nature is this higher truth.

Though stillness is your connection to your higher truth, that stillness is not your higher truth. You, as your higher truth, are the one that is aware of your thoughts, physical body, and all that you experience, including the stillness. The essential aspect of who you are is beyond your ability to experience. The fundamental aspect of who you are is aware of all of experience. You are multidimensional being as your essential being is beyond experience while simultaneously manifesting as a physical being that is intended for experience.

Quantum physics has provided scientific evidence that we are multi-dimensional beings. We can use a brick as an example. When we look at a brick, we see a solid object that has shape, size, and weight. If we had the ability to look at the brick at the atomic level, we would see atoms separated by vast distances of space. This phrase is not entirely accurate since even atoms are not solid, they are fluctuations of energy. At the essential and most fundamental level, a brick is fluctuations of energy and the vastness of space. At this level, there is no sense of separation or distinction between the brick and the world around it. At this level, there is only oneness.

We have forgotten our higher truth, which I refer to as consciousness, because we have identified with body and mind. In other words, we define ourselves by our thoughts and physical body. Because we define ourselves as a physical body with thoughts, we experience ourselves as being separate from others, our environment, and our higher truth.

That we see ourselves as being separate from consciousness is no mistake. It is a necessary aspect for the expansion of consciousness. Consciousness is like the atomic level of the brick. There is only oneness. To expand, consciousness needs to experience itself. To experience itself, consciousness needs to experience separation. You and I and every living and non-living being are the physical manifestations of consciousness. By taking on a physical manifestation, there comes a sense of separation, and with separation arises the feeling of contrast. The only way you can know that you have a weight problem is by comparing yourself to someone else.

The thoughts and feelings that you experience when comparing yourself to others allow consciousness to experience itself by way of this information. Upon experiencing itself, consciousness creates conditions that are consistent with how it experiences itself. These conditions become your experience as the manifested self. If you believe that due to your weight problem, you are undesirable, consciousness will manifest the conditions that reinforce or support that belief. This dynamic between your manifest self and consciousness is referred to as the Law of Attraction.

But this is who I am!

As indicated earlier, you took on your manifested self for the purpose of being able to experience; however, just manifesting as a physical form is not enough to experience. There is also a need for a sense of separation. Only when there is a sense of "I" can there be a sense of other. That sense of "I," known as the ego, is what creates a sense of separation. With a sense of separation arises a feeling of contrast, and it is from contrast that experience is created. The reason why the human species has been able to achieve its current level of technology and has had such an impact on this planet is due to our identifying ourselves with our experiences.

While other life forms have a sense of "I," that sense of "I" is not identified with the physical form or thought. A dog has a sense of "I," but this sense of "I" does not identify itself with the dog's physical form or thoughts. The dog has an awareness of its sense of "I" and its experiences, but it does not self-identify with its experiences. Dogs do not develop a self-image of being overweight or unattractive, which we do.

To better understand how experience and self-identification affect our lives, imagine the following two scenarios. Jon is like 95% of the rest of humanity in that his sense of self is largely determined by external circumstances. Being toned, athletic, and fit, Jon's physical appearance is a great sense of pride for him as he knows that he looks good. Jon also has a highly paid job that allows him to live a luxurious lifestyle, which only adds to his sense of feeling good about himself.

The challenge for Jon is that his sense of self is not permanent. Rather, it is in constant flux. While Jon's physical conditioning and career success make him feel good about himself, Jon often experiences the fear of not being good enough when his feelings of insecurity appear. These feelings occur when he is reminded of how he felt as a child when he felt invalidated by his parents. He also experiences a sense of doubt as to his sense of desirability when he sees others getting more attention than he is.

Jon's sense of self is object-oriented, meaning that it depends on his body, career, memories, and how others are responding to him.

Most of us are like Jon because we have lost touch with our higher truth. We are suffering amnesia and have forgotten who we are at the most fundamental level. Everything that we experience is impermanent. Nothing is in the phenomenal world lasts. Physical shape, financial success, and how others respond to us will change. The word "phenomena" refers to something that we can detect using our five senses or something we can experience from within. For this reason, thoughts and feelings are also always changing. Whenever we base our sense of self on that which is impermanent, we experience suffering.

The second scenario involves you, the reader. Remember the exercise that you did at the beginning of this chapter? If you do not remember your experience of that activity, please repeat it. While you were experiencing that stillness, did you feel a sense peace or calmness? Did you think of your past or the future? I know your answer to this question if you experienced that stillness. The answer was no! The reason why you feel stillness and calm was because you were connecting with your higher truth, or consciousness. Unlike the phenomenal world, your higher truth, or consciousness, is independent of anything that you can experience. It is eternal and cannot be touched by anything that you could ever experience.

When we base our life on this, you will not need to learn about the Law of Attraction, nor will you have to worry about weight loss. You will accomplish all of your desires effortlessly. We will explore the reasons for this in the next chapter.

Falling Back into the Rhythm of Life

"If you hear a voice within you say 'you cannot paint,' then by all means, paint, and that voice will be silenced."

-Vincent Van Gogh

In the previous chapter, we discussed three important points that we need to keep in mind to understand the significance of this section. The three points are:

- You are a multi-dimensional being in that your essence is nonphysical while at the same time manifesting as a physical being.
- You experience yourself as physical being for the purpose of experiencing contrast.
- Through contrast, you gain information, which leads to the expansion of consciousness both at your manifested and unmanifested level.

The following is an example of these three points. The purpose of consciousness is to expand, but expansion requires information. To gain information about itself, the larger consciousness manifests as a physical from named Mary. As the greater consciousness, Mary only has an awareness of herself, the larger consciousness. As a physical manifestation, Mary experiences herself as a physical being that is separate from other manifested entities, which allows her to experience contrast.

Mary takes a walk in the park one day and comes across an attractive woman. This lady is vibrant and active, which Mary admires. She sees this woman playing a game of soccer with her male friends. Mary experiences thoughts of how happy and fortunate this woman is while comparing herself to this woman, which is the experience of contrast. Mary's experience of contrast leads to Mary having thoughts about herself and the other woman. The thoughts that Mary experiences create her emotions. The thoughts and emotions that Mary experiences become a source of information for the larger consciousness.

As indicated earlier, the greater consciousness is only aware of itself, which is oneness without any sense of separation or differentiation. Mary's thoughts and emotions provide the larger consciousness with new information that allows it to experience itself as the new information. Since it is the purpose of consciousness to expand, the greater consciousness will take Mary's information and manifest as those beings or conditions that are similar to the information that it received.

If the thoughts Mary had about the other woman were "See is so beautiful and fit. She is so unlike me. I am just a fat nobody," these thought leads to the generation of emotions such as sadness, resentment, or hurt.

As the larger consciousness experiences itself as these thoughts and feelings, which are all forms of energy, it will manifest those conditions that match this information. These manifested conditions will continue to appear in Mary's life for her to experience.

As long as Mary continues to interpret her experience with the same kind of thinking, Mary's experience of herself will not change. It is important to note that the larger consciousness, or the universe, completely lacks any form of judgment. It is only responding to the information that it receives from us.

Now let us imagine a different scenario where Mary experiences thoughts of a different quality when seeing the other woman. This time, Mary's thoughts of the other woman are, "She is so beautiful and in such great shape. I admire her.

That's it! I am ready to change how I live my life." This kind of thinking leads to the emotions of excitement, determination, and happiness. The larger consciousness will experience itself in this manner and manifest in Mary's life those conditions that support this information. It is this manifestation process that is known as the Law of Attraction. Our thoughts and feelings are the key factors that determine what we attract in our lives. The next three sections will discuss thoughts, beliefs, emotions, and feelings in greater depth.

Reflections of the Universe

"The key to change... is to let go of fear."

-Rosanne Cash

As multi-dimensional beings, we may have developed amnesia when it comes to recognizing ourselves as being consciousness. However, our direct connection with that consciousness is impossible to ignore. Our thoughts, feelings, and emotions provide a vital feedback system that allows us to tap into the larger consciousness while at the same time creating our experience. By developing an understanding of our thoughts, feelings, and emotions, we can tap into greater levels of our human potential, which is unlimited.

Thoughts

Earlier in this book, we discussed how we self-identify with our minds and bodies. As for the mind, we believe that the thoughts we experience are ours, that we are ones that are doing the thinking, and that we are the creator of our thoughts. From higher levels of awareness, it becomes evident that we are not separate, independent beings from the rest of life. Think of the earlier example of the brick, which appears solid from our perspective, but is indistinguishable from the surrounding space at the atomic level.

Our relationship to the larger consciousness commonly referred to as the universe is also dependent on our perspective. From the plane of ordinary awareness, we are separate from our experiences of each other and the world around us. From the viewpoint of higher levels of consciousness, we realize that each one of us is inseparable from the universe. In fact, what we call the universe is consciousness expressing itself as many forms. You and consciousness, or the universe, are no more separate from each other than an ocean current is distinct from the ocean.

Rather than being the one that thinks thoughts, your manifested being is tapping into the thoughts of the larger consciousness. Your mind is like a cell phone tower that picks up the signal from a satellite. Every thought that has ever been thought, or will be thought, is part of the information and energy field that makes up the larger consciousness. Rather than having a thought, you are accessing that thought. The more that we identify our thoughts, the less we will be able to tap into that informational energy field.

People who have ESP, clairvoyance, out of body experiences, and other psychic abilities, can do so because they can tap into this field. They can relax their minds enough to lose their attachments or self-identification with it, which is often accomplished through meditation.

The thoughts that you attract are pure information and lack any inherent power. What gives thoughts their power is the attention that we give them. You have thousands of thoughts every day. Only a small fraction of these thoughts appear in your awareness. The thoughts that arise in your awareness do so because you make them meaningful. If we do not make our thoughts important, they will often pass through our consciousness largely unnoticed. When we have a conviction that a thought is true, that thought becomes a belief.

Our beliefs are compelling, so powerful that they drive every aspect of our lives. Our beliefs determine what we focus on, what we overlook, what we are willing to do, what we will avoid, our relationships with others, and how we experience the world. We can think of our beliefs as tinted sunglasses. If you are wearing sunglasses that are tinted blue, everything you experience will appear to be blue. If a person believes that they are undesirable because of their weight, that belief will determine what that person focuses on, what they are oblivious of, who they associate with, how they live their life, and how they perceive others and themselves.

Just as with thoughts, beliefs lack any inherent power of their own. Our beliefs are energized by the amount of attention we give them. Our beliefs rely on us to obtain their power, which leads to an important point. Your beliefs are neither true nor false, nor do they reflect reality. Rather, our beliefs create our reality!

In 1954, the world speed record for running a mile was broken by Roger Bannister, who ran a mile in less than four minutes. Before Bannister, no runner had ever run a mile under four minutes. Since Bannister's record achievement, many other runners have run a mile under four minutes, so many, in fact, that Bannister's running time became a new standard for other runners.

Why is it that no runner completed the mile run in less than four minutes before Bannister's achievement? Why is it that so many runners have beaten Bannister's record since then? The answer to these questions is the power of belief. Bannister's achievement showed other runners that it was possible. Until Bannister, it was believed that running a mile in less than four minutes was not feasible.

Our beliefs are a demonstration of the Law of Attraction working. When we energize a thought by focusing our awareness on it, that thought attracts other thoughts of similar quality, just as a magnet attracts iron filings. A person may have the thought, "I am overweight." By repeatedly giving this thought their attention, it becomes energized and starts to attract other thoughts such as:

- "I need to diet."
- "I am unattractive."
- "I am a pig."
- "I need to lose weight."
- "I have always failed to lose weight."
- "Diets never work."

Any thought that is attracted to the original thought "I am overweight" becomes the potential target of our attention. If this occurs, it will also become energized and attract other thoughts like "I guess I was born this way," or "I need to join a health club." It is this process that creates a belief.

The Most Powerful Thought in the Universe

In the previous section, an example of how beliefs are created was given, and that process started with the person having the thought, "I am overweight." It was also explained that a thought that is energized attracts other thoughts.

Given this, what was the thought that attracted the thought "I am overweight?" The answer to this question is the most powerful thought in the universe. That thought is "I." Every living being manifests in this world with the knowledge that "I exist" or "I am." We have given this thought so much attention that any thought that becomes attracted to it becomes part of our sense of identity, including our thoughts on our mind and body. The thought "I am overweight," occurs when the "I" thought attracts the thought "overweight" through the power of attention.

Why do some people energize the thought "overweight," while others do not? Conditioning determines this. Russian physiologist Ivan Pavlov did a famous experiment where he presented a piece of meat to a dog while at the same time ringing a bell. The first time that he did this, the dog was interested only in the food and had no interest in the sound. Before giving the dog the meat, the dog would salivate in anticipation.

Pavlov repeated this experiment over and over until all he had to do was ring the bell and the dog would salivate upon hearing it, even though there was no meat being offered. The dog had learned to associate the sound of the bell with food. The reason why our "I" thought attracts the "overweight" thought is that we have been conditioned to associate this thought with the perception that we have of ourselves. It is the beliefs that we attach to the thought "overweight" that determines what being overweight means to us.

The belief that we have for being overweight is the result of conditioning and is based on how we were raised and the norms of society. It is no surprise that the children of overweight parents are frequently overweight themselves. The beliefs of the parents have impacted how they have raised their children. If the parents use food as a way to deal with the fears and insecurities that they have, their children will adopt the same beliefs. The parents' habitual dietary habits will also be imposed on their children.

That which determines the meaning that we give to being overweight is also determined by society and culture. Americans have a negative association toward being overweight while there are other parts of the world where being overweight is accepted.

Whether we are accepting of being overweight or shamed by it, we limit ourselves when define ourselves by it. When we identify with our minds and body, the "I" thought takes on the tinted sunglasses of that thought. It is for this reason that most people find weight loss difficult. By identifying with the thought "I am overweight," we have developed a sense of resistance toward ourselves, which we will discuss in more detail in a later chapter.

Feelings and Emotions

As noted a few times earlier, everything arises from consciousness, and that by manifesting in physical form, we can experience contrast and gain information for the expanding of consciousness. Thoughts are a form of energy that manifests as phenomenal form. The word "phenomenal" refers to an object that can be experienced by our five senses or in our awareness. Though we cannot detect a thought using our five senses, we are aware of their existence as long as we do not suppress them in our subconscious. When thoughts are contained in our subconscious, we lack awareness of them. Even though subconscious thoughts avoid our detection, they never the less impact our lives. One of the reasons why many people have trouble losing weight is because the thoughts that are driving their behavior to eat in an unhealthy way are frequently subconscious. We have been provided with a powerful tool to detect the thoughts that we are experiencing, be they conscious or not, and that tool is our emotions. Our emotions are the mirror of our mind. They are the tangible signals that indicate the quality of thoughts that we are experiencing.

When we have negative or disempowering thoughts, we experience emotions of like kind. The feelings of anger, fear, resentment, and jealousy are a reflection of thoughts of the same nature, just as are the emotions of love, compassion, joy, gratitude, and appreciation are the reflection of thoughts of the same kind. If we ever want to understand what we are thinking, all we need to do is pay attention to the emotions that we are experiencing.

Our feelings can be arranged in a hierarchy based on their energetic level. Shame has the lowest energy level, followed by the emotions of guilt, apathy, grief, and fear, in that order. Moving more toward the center of the hierarchy are desire, anger, and pride. These emotions are considered higher than the low-end emotions because they have a higher energy level, which is more likely to lead us to take some form of action.

Moving toward the upper end of the hierarchy are courage, gratitude, appreciation, joy, and love, which is the highest level of emotion. These emotions are considered to be higher level because they cause us to move beyond our sense of separation and self-identification with the ego and place a greater focus on others. It is for this reason that the emotion of appreciation has a higher vibration than that of gratitude. Normally, when we experience a sense of gratitude, it is the result of us receiving something from another person or because we recognize the value of something that we have. The emotion of appreciation is a higher vibration because we can experience it without any reference to ourselves, as in the case of the appreciation of a beautiful sunset.

The more consistently we can maintain the higher level of emotions, the more effective we will be in attracting that which we desire since we can only attract into our lives that which matches the level of vibration that we are experiencing. When we are experiencing unconditional love, our love is at the highest vibratory level.

We experience unconditional love when we learn to replace any sense of resistance with a spirit of acceptance, especially self-acceptance. When I say acceptance, I do not mean that we tolerate or agree with conditions that we find unsatisfactory. Rather, we accept things the way they are by not being resistant to them. Only when we fully accept our circumstances can we focus on improving them. As long as we express resistance to our current reality, we will continue to attract into our lives those people, objects, and situations that reflect our resistance.

The Unseen Power of Resistance

We live in a society that thrives on resistance, which is why so many people are unfulfilled. We are unfulfilled because we are caught between two powerful forces, one of which is manufactured and propagated by our species while the other is the power of the universe seeking wholeness.

Most of the human race has lost touch with their connection to the larger consciousness. They experience themselves as a mind and body that are separate from the rest of the world. We have learned to define ourselves by our thoughts, actions, and physical being. Since we are raised within a culture or society, we judge ourselves based on the established norms of that society or culture.

When our sense of identity is consistent with the established criteria, we feel acceptance for ourselves. However, this feeling of acceptance is very rare and usually found within the context of indigenous people who are relatively isolated from the modern world. Most of us have been raised in large societies that are entrenched in laws, rules, regulations, commercialism, and diverse viewpoints.

We are always adapting our thinking and behavior to meet the expectations of our family, societal standards, and the mass media. Take time to consider the expectations that you are bombarded by as they relate to weight. How does your family view those who are overweight? What is the message that you get from the self-help industry regarding being overweight? What do the media and society tell you about being overweight? Is the message that you get loving and supportive, or is it judgmental?

Now let us compare our experiences of conforming to the societal expectations to the force that is the universe, a force that imbues our manifested self and guides us toward a sense of wholeness. Before we discuss this in greater detail, let us explore an aspect of our lives that we all can relate to, which is deep sleep. Do you enjoy deep sleep? I am going to assume your response would be, "Yes!" I want you to think about what it is like while you are in a deep sleep. Are you having any difficulty doing this? No problem, no one can.

When we are in a deep sleep, we are liberated from all of our thoughts. By liberating ourselves from our thoughts, we are devoid of any sense of experience, including our experience of ourselves. Remember that we manifested as physical beings for the purpose of experiencing and experiencing requires contrast. Without thoughts, there is no contrast. Without contrast, there is no sense of separation. Without separation, there is wholeness. We love deep sleep because we experience a sense of wholeness. In deep sleep, we lose all sense of personal identity. Without a sense of personal identity, there is nothing to conform to or expectations of how we need to be. When we enter deep sleep, we return to the larger consciousness, our unmanifested self.

We have just explored the two powerful forces, the force of society and our attempts to conform to it to feel accepted, and the force that is your true nature which is guiding you to return to wholeness. Every challenge or problem that you have ever faced, or will ever face, is the result of us trying to gain acceptance within society and its artificial standards while forgetting the eternal aspect of ourselves, which is established in wholeness. Anytime we choose society over our natural being, we experience ourselves as being fragmented.

Any sense of resistance that we experience within ourselves is due to us feeling fragmented. We feel fragmented because we have bought into societies expectations. When we do not meet those expectations, we declare war on that part of ourselves that does not fit those expectations, such as being overweight.

Every self-help product, self-improvement resource, and dieting program either explicitly or indirectly points to the fact that we are not good enough the way we are; that we need to change something about ourselves to become happy. If we are trying to lose weight so that we can feel better about ourselves, what we are saying is that our body is not sufficient and that it has become an obstacle to us in our pursuit of feeling happy. Because it is a barrier, we develop a sense of resistance to it.

When we resist anything in life, it means that we become vigilant of it. In other words, we focus on it. When we place our attention on being overweight, we usually experience a disempowering emotion such as guilt, shame, hopelessness, or anger. This most subtle and seemingly innocent act of placing our attention on being overweight and feeling negative emotions activates the Law of Attraction to manifest all the conditions that are consistent with the energy level of that emotion. This is why most people struggle to lose weight. They are sending a message to the universe to fill their lives with all things that make losing weight a struggle. The struggle has nothing to do with losing weight; it is because we are expecting one thing but telling the universe that we want something else.

Feelings

Before discussing feelings, let us do a quick review. Thoughts are forms of energy that we tap into. We do not think thoughts, rather, we access thoughts by attracting them. Like everything else in this universe, thoughts are just forms of energy. The kind of thoughts we attract depends on the vibrational level of our lives, and the energy level of our lives can be determined by the emotions we are experiencing. I stated earlier that emotions are a mirror of our thoughts. What is more accurate is that our emotions are a reflection of our thoughts because the quality of our emotions determines the quality of the thoughts we attract.

The thoughts we attract are not original thoughts. In fact, there are no original thoughts. Rather, there is a storehouse of thoughts, and that repository contains every thought that was ever thought or will ever be thought. In this respect, we recycle thoughts from this storehouse, which is sometimes referred to as the Akashic records or the collective consciousness. You and I can tap into the same thoughts that were experienced by Jesus, the Buddha, your best friend, or a dog.

As an energy form, feelings are different from thoughts in that they are purer than thoughts. Feelings are unique to you and the larger consciousness. We can think of feelings as being signals that inform us on how aligned we are with the greater consciousness. Whenever we experience feelings of well-being, we are aware that we are in alignment with our highest self or the universe. Whenever we are experiencing feelings that are not consistent with wellbeing, we know that we are out of alignment with our highest self.

You can think of your feelings as your GPS to the larger consciousness. You are on course to arrive at a sense of wholeness when you live your life in a manner that feels right to you. When we subordinate our feelings and live our lives per the expectations of others, we, of course, experience suffering. No one can provide you with the answers as to how to live your life or how to become happy because each one of us has manifested on this planet with our very own unique purpose. It is only through honoring our feelings that we can discover that purpose.

The challenge is that most of us are not in touch with our emotions, or if we are, we often blur the line between what we feel and think. My message to you is this: From the perspective of higher levels of consciousness, you will never find happiness if you become a slave to your thoughts. Your thoughts will never bring you the experience of peace, wellbeing, or higher levels of awareness. Nor will you ever lose the weight that you desire if you follow the dictates of your mind. Our thoughts are necessary for problem-solving everyday situations, but beyond that, your thoughts will only drive you crazy. If you want to lose weight, you need to get in touch with your feelings and follow your GPS.

Weight Loss Through the Use of the Law of Attraction

"Change your thoughts, and you change your world."

-Norman Vincent Peale

Losing weight through the use of the Law of Attraction is no different than attracting anything else thing that you desire. What is most important is for you to prepare yourself so that you can manifest that which you desire: losing weight. Before we discuss how to use the Law of Attraction to lose weight, it is important to briefly address a few common misunderstandings regarding the Law of Attraction.

The first thing to point out is that you do not need to learn how to use the Law of Attraction because you are using it already. In fact, it is impossible for you not to manifest. You are always manifesting, but you may not be aware of it. Remember, what we attract is based on our energy level, which we can identify by the emotions that we experience.

We may want to draw the conditions that lead us to lose weight, but if we harbor any doubt about our ability to manifest, or if we hold subconscious beliefs about ourselves that are disempowering, the universe will get a mixed message. Given that our subconscious beliefs and doubt are often stronger than our conscious intent, we do not get the results that we desire. In this section of the book, you will discuss practical ways to uncover your subconscious beliefs, reduce any resistance that you may have, raise your sense of certainty, and most important of all, simple ways to cultivate greater love and acceptance for yourself. In fact, by developing greater love and acceptance for yourself, everything else in your life will fall into place by itself.

Gaining greater self-love and self-acceptance is the most powerful thing you can do to employ the Law of Attraction effectively. In fact, self-love and self-acceptance are the most powerful things that you can do to lose weight. By developing greater self-love and self-acceptance, you will raise your energy levels, develop greater self-awareness, and lower your level of resistance, all of which lead to enhanced manifesting ability and healthier living.

Before we launch into the exercises, I would like to share with you an important observation. If you go out into nature, you will find wild animals and plants living out their lives. At no time will you find a wild animal that is overweight or out of shape. You will not find any animals that are attempting to meet the expectations of other animals. Nor you will find any animals trying to improve themselves. The same thing can be said of plants; you will not find any plants that are exerting themselves to become better plants.

What separates us from the rest of nature is that other living beings live their life by following the rhythms of life and nature's wisdom. All living and nonliving beings are manifestations of consciousness. However, they have maintained their connection to it. There was no need for other living beings to develop the way our species did because they have maintained their connection to their source. While we are gifted as a species in our ability for self-reflection and high intelligence, we have limited ourselves from experiencing our higher potentials and wellness of being because our ego has left us with a sense of separation and the illusions that we are somehow flawed.

While we claim to be the most intelligent and successful species on the planet, we engage in widespread destructive behaviors, behaviors that are destructive to others, toward the environment, and toward ourselves. Overeating is just one example of this kind of destruction. The biggest obstacle in losing weight is our egos. Our egos lead us to compare ourselves to others. Our egos tell us that we are not good enough and cause us to blame others for the difficulties that we experience.

For most people, losing weight does not require special diets or pills. Special diets and pills do not address the cause of being overweight, which is that we have lost our balance with the wisdom of nature. No animal goes on a diet; they just live their lives in tune with nature's greater wisdom. You and I are no different. To live with self-love and self-acceptance is to live by nature's wisdom, and nature's wisdom is the Law of Attraction.

The Role of Resistance and Weight Loss

Every one of us has done something that we did not want to do. We agreed to do a favor for a friend when we did not want to. We attended a social event when we wanted to stay home and have a quiet evening. Or we ate something with too many calories and felt guilty afterward. The first two examples illustrated how we are resistant to doing something but do it anyway, while the third example demonstrates how we did what we wanted to do but then created resistance toward ourselves after the fact.

Anytime we do things begrudgingly, we are creating a misalignment in our life. Anytime we do something willingly but feel guilty about it afterward, we are creating a misalignment in our life. You may take pause regarding my last statement, after all, isn't guilt healthy in some cases? "If I harm another person, shouldn't I feel guilty?" Of course! From the perspective of everyday consciousness, this is what is expected. However, to effectively use the Law of Attraction, you need to enter higher levels of consciousness.

From the perspective of everyday consciousness, I cause harm to another person and then feel guilty about it, which inflicts damage on me. Feeling guilty may make me think twice before remaking the same mistake. However, this type of thinking is just part of the socialization process that we have bought into. If we harmed another person, it was due to the pain that we were experiencing within ourselves. When we feel guilty, we are adding to the pain that we were already experiencing. As our experience of pain means that we are out of alignment with our higher self, guilt just increases our lack of alignment. If you are overweight, it is not an issue of too many calories; it is because you are subconsciously trying to dull the pain of being out of alignment.

When we achieve greater conscious awareness, we improve our alignment. When we enhance our alignment, we will experience a greater sense of peace and well-being. Thus, we are less likely to cause harm to others. We will less likely cause harm to others because we have a greater level of awareness to the thoughts, emotions, and feelings that we are experiencing, and we are less likely to personalize them, making us less reactive during emotional situations. Should we harm others, we can address the situation with a greater level of compassion for both them and ourselves. Because we have compassion for ourselves and the other person, guilt is not needed, and we preserve our alignment, which can only benefit those around us. Finally, because we have compassion, there is no reason to overeat as we are emotionally aware.

We have covered a lot of information so far in this book, and I suspect some of you may find what has been written sounds abstract or difficult to understand. You may even question my comments that the essence of who we are is consciousness or the practicality of using the Law of Attraction to lose weight. Whatever you may believe, go with it. Do not try to understand that which has been written. I say this because, in a way, I have undertaken an impossible task in writing this book. I say this because I am using words and concepts to explain that which cannot be explained. That which I have written about is beyond the grasps of the mind to understand.

The words in this book are no more than pointers to a larger truth, a truth that can only be understood through directly experiencing it. This is why I say do not get so caught up in trying to understand that which I have written. Rather, allow yourself to absorb this information based on where you are in your conscious development. I had gone to the level of detail that I have because I wanted you to get the "big picture" of what causes us to gain weight. Allow me to take all that I have written so far and restate it in a more relatable manner.

Regardless of the problems that we may be experiencing, be it weight issues or anything else, the problem that we are facing is not the cause of our suffering. Rather, it is us identifying with our problems that create suffering. When we identify with the problem, we lose touch with the truth of who we are. It is not the problems in life that get us; it is how we define our relationship with them. Some people are entering the sunset of their lives and are experiencing a level of gratitude, appreciation, and inner peace that they have never experienced before.

Some mothers have not only forgiven the murderers of their children but are actively involved in supporting them in creating a new direction for their lives. Some people risk their lives as they respond to the needs of a stranger. Whether the people in these examples are aware of it or not, they have based their lives on something greater than any fear that they may experience.

Can you trust your life over any perceived fear that may come from societal standards or your imagination? Can you trust that the cause of your weight problem has little to do with what you eat, but more with the relationship that you have with yourself? How do you develop this kind of trust in your life? You do it through self-love. Learning to love yourself is not being narcissistic or self-absorbed, rather, to love yourself is to contribute to the saving of this planet. The only reason why war, violence, social injustice, and the destruction of the environment exist is that we do not love ourselves. Because we do not love ourselves, we focus on the fear in our lives and view the world around us as a threat.

Throughout this book, I have made reference to the larger consciousness. This term "larger consciousness" is just another name for love. Love is wholeness, connection, and the lack of separation or distinction. To be an enlightened being is to understand your connection to the larger consciousness, which is love. To be an enlightened being is to love yourself, just the way you are at this moment, regardless of your history. To have self-love is to practice the Law of Attraction effectively, whether you are doing it intentionally or not.

The remaining part of this section contains exercises for accessing self-love. I use the word "accessing" instead of "developing" self-love because there is nothing to improve. The essence of who you are is love; you just need to learn to step out of its way. The same is true with practicing the Law of Attraction or reaching your desired weight. Life will take care of these things for you if you just learn to trust it and just follow its guidance. The exercises are divided into three groups:

- The first group involves uncovering your hidden beliefs and changing them.
- The second group contains meditative exercises to help you increase your awareness to the nature of your mind and body.
- The activities in the third group involve using what you learned in the first two groups and using that information to make transformations in your life. It is these changes that will put you in alignment to effectively use the Law of Attraction.

Group 1

As we discussed earlier, our beliefs are the organizing principles for how we experience life. It is essential that you recognize beliefs that are disempowering you to become effective manifesters. Additionally, our beliefs are directly linked to our weight issues. By identifying the beliefs that create resistance in our lives, we bring them to the light of our awareness where they lose their potency. We then can then develop new and more empowering beliefs to take their place. The very process of identifying our disempowering beliefs and adopting empowering ones is an act of self-love.

The Ultimate Why

With sincere reflection, most of us can determine why we do the things that we do. However, what we get is usually just a surface answer. If we want to get to the cause of what drives our thinking or behavior, we need to reveal the ultimate why, which is subconscious. If we are overeating, it is because we are using food as a way to comfort ourselves and distract us from the cause. In this exercise, you will identify the underlying belief, or beliefs, which you have allowed to slip from your awareness.

Before you start the exercise, take the time to write down those aspects of your life that are bothering you. When you make your list, it is important to be brutally honest with yourself. Do not hold anything back.

When you have made your list, determine which of these items most impacts the way you feel about yourself. You will be using this item for the exercise. For the purpose of this exercise, I will use an example so that you can see how the process works. The problem I chose was: "I feel angry that my husband is always criticizing me."

1. Once you have written out the problem, you want to ask, "What does it mean to me to have my husband criticize me?"

2. My answer would be, "It means that he does not understand me."

3. I would then ask myself, "What does it mean to me to have my husband not understand me?"

4. I would respond by saying, "It means that I made a mistake in marrying him."

5. I would then ask, "What does it mean to me to have made a mistake in marrying him?"

6. I would respond, "That it is just another example of how I have screwed my life up, that I cannot do anything right."

7. I would then ask, "What does screwing my life up and not doing anything right mean to me?"

8. I would respond with, "It means that I am hopeless and that I am not good enough."

9. I would then ask, "What does it mean to be hopeless and not good enough?"

10. I would respond with "It means that no one will ever love me."

The belief that "No one will ever love me" is the cause, the root belief that causing my suffering. Believing that my husband criticizes me is just an expression of my root belief that I am projecting that idea on his behavior and making him the cause of my problems. If a perfect stranger criticized me, it would create little impact on me because I have no attachments to the stranger. Given that I have strong attachments to my husband, his criticisms take on a whole new dimension. In fact, how other act toward me, regardless of who they are, would be of little consequence to me if I were established in my connection to myself through self-love.

Without identifying the root belief of my suffering, I would turn to food to distract myself from the feelings. A lack of awareness of this root belief allows it to express itself in its full strength and energetic level. Since this belief was subconscious, I was unaware of its influence on my life and how it was attracting unwanted conditions into my life. This is why so many people get mixed results, if any, when employing the Law of Attraction. They are only aware of their conscious intent but are blind to their root belief. It is the lack of awareness of this root belief that prevents most people from losing weight permanently. Their diets, pills, or exercises may shed the pounds, but their root belief will cause them to return to behaviors that do not support them in their happiness.

Turning the Tables on a Root Belief

Now that you have identified your root belief, your next step is to reprogram your brain by identifying with all the pain that your root belief has caused you and all the benefits you would gain by abandoning it and replacing it with an empowering belief. To do this exercise, do the following:

1. Get two sheets of paper. Select paper sizes 8" x 11" or larger.

2. Take the first piece of paper and fold it in half lengthwise.

3. On the top of the paper, write down your root belief.

4. Make a list on the left-hand side of the paper of all the ways this belief has cost you in your life. When doing this part of the exercise, think of how this root belief has affected you in all areas of your life. Ask yourself how this belief has affected you in the way you see yourself, how it has affected your emotional health, relationships, physical health, work, finances, and so on.

5. When writing, keep in mind the following:

   • When writing this list, write down the first thing that comes to your mind, even if it seems irrelevant.

   • Write as fast as you can and feel the emotions that arise. This is a heartfelt exercise, not a thinking one.

   • Keep writing until you run out of things to write.

6. Beside each item that you write down, assign an arbitrary point value as to how much impact this item has had on you. When selecting the point value, choose the first number that comes to mind.

7. When you have completed assigning the point values, find the total of all the point values and place it at the bottom of the page.

8. For the right side of the page, repeat Steps 6-7, except this time, you will write down all the ways that this belief has benefited you.

When you have completed Step 8, think of a new alternative belief that empowers you. For example, if the original belief was, "No one will ever love me," the new belief might be, "The only love that I can depend on is the love that I give to myself."

On the second paper, repeat steps 1-8 using your new belief with the following exceptions: Reverse Steps 6 and 8 by writing down all the ways that you believe that you would benefit from this new belief for Step 6. When doing Step 8, write down all the ways you think it will cost you.

When you have completed the two sheets, do the following:

1. Immediately review your lists, allowing yourself to experience any emotions that arise.

2. Review yours lists every day, once in the morning and once before you go to bed, until you become fully associated with the emotions that you experience.

When you become fully associated with the costs of holding onto your old belief with the benefits of adopting your new belief, your mind will become programmed with your new belief.

The following is an alternative to the last exercise for changing your beliefs and involves meditation:

1. On the piece of paper, write down a belief that you have which limits you or is causing you unhappiness.

2. When you have written down the belief, sit in a comfortable position and close your eyes.

3. Allow yourself to follow your breath during inhalation and exhalation. Place your attention on your breath. Feel it as it courses through your body. Relax.

4. I want you to think of the belief that you wrote down. Feel the heaviness and weight that this belief has had on your life.

5. What has been the cost to your happiness for holding this belief? Can you think of specific instances? Did this belief cost you a relationship? If so, who is no longer in your life because of this belief?

6. Has this belief cost you money? Did this belief lead you to engage in risky behavior with your money or health? What about your sense of self?

7. How has this belief affected your self-confidence or self-esteem? Take the time to feel the pain that this belief has created for your life.

8. Allow yourself to experience it fully, experience the emotions and feelings that come with living with this belief.

9. How will this belief affect your future? If you continue to hold on to this belief, what will your life be like a year from now, five years from now, and 15 years from now? See your life in the future. What consequences will you experience if you continue to maintain this belief?

10. As mentioned before, thoughts and beliefs do not have any power other than the power we give them. Unto themselves, our thoughts and beliefs lack any power. Our beliefs are not true or untrue, they just exist. It is us who grant them power over our lives.

11. Now open your eyes and get your writing instrument. This negative belief you just meditated on existed because you perceived in your mind that there was a benefit to having this belief.

12. Write down what why you believe that you adopted this belief. For example, if you have a belief that you cannot depend on or trust other people, the benefit of this belief may be that it protected you from getting hurt.

13. Now think of a belief that will offer the same benefit without creating limitations for you. Using the previous example, a new belief could be, "I can trust others because I am learning to trust myself." Write down your new belief.

14. When you have written down the belief, sit down in a comfortable position and close your eyes.

15. Allow yourself to follow your breath during inhalation and exhalation. Place your attention on your breath. Feel it as it courses through your body. Relax.

16. I want you to think of the new belief that you wrote down. Think about what your life would be like if you operated from this new belief from this moment on.

17. How would living with this new belief make you feel about yourself? How would it impact those that you care about? What would your life be like? Think about what your life would be like one year from now if you started to live by this new belief today. What do you think it would be like five years from now?

18. As you think about what your life would be like, allow yourself to experience the emotions and feelings that arise. Allow yourself to sink into these emotions and feelings. You may want to visualize yourself acting from this new belief.

19. Practice this meditation every day for three weeks, which is how long it typically takes to create a habit. The mind cannot tell the difference between visualization and doing. Meditating regularly will reprogram your subconscious, leading you to take the appropriate action.

Putting your Words into Action

Now that you have turned the tables on your beliefs, I want you to make a list of all the actions that you could take that would be consistent with your new belief. Using my example "The only love that I can depend on is the love that I give to myself," I would think of all the ways that I could express love to myself. Many people have problems with this exercise because they overthink. This exercise is very easy. Simply think of all things that give you a sense of pleasure or enjoyment. Make your list as long as possible and make a commitment that you will do at least one of the items on your list each day. By taking action on your new belief, your new belief will be strengthened.

Group 2

Now that you have started the process of cultivating your new empowering belief, it is time to challenge the most fundamental perceptions that you hold for yourself and the world around you. These are contemplative exercises, meaning that mediation is involved. If you have never meditated before, do not be concerned. Meditation is simple. In fact, it is beyond easy; it means exerting no effort. Instead, meditation involves the embracing and total acceptance of that which you are experiencing. Any problems that you may encounter when trying to meditate are the result of the mental habits that you have engaged in for most of your life. We will start with a simple exercise and work toward more challenging activities. I recommend you practice each exercise until you are comfortable with it before progressing. My intent in offering you these exercises is to get you to question yourself as to how you have perceived your life and the world around you. We engage in overeating and other unhealthy habits because we have bought into erroneous perceptions of the world which cause us to identify with our mind and body overly.

Basic Meditation

1. Find a quiet place to sit that is comfortable. You may sit on the floor or in a chair.

2. Close your eyes and allow yourself to relax by putting your attention on the flow of your breath. Keep your awareness on your breath as you inhale by focusing on the sensations of your breath during inhalation. Do the same thing during exhalation by experiencing the feelings that are experienced as your breath travels out of your body. Breathe naturally; it is important that you make no effort at any time during this meditation. An alternative to following your breath is to observe the rising and falling of your abdomen.

3. As you breathe, you will experience thoughts, perceptions, and sensations. They will have different qualities to them. Some will be pleasant while others may be uncomfortable or even frightening. Regardless of what you experience, do not interfere with them. Do not try to control, change, or analyze them. Become a scientist who is committed only to observing them.

4. Anytime you catch your mind wandering, just return your attention to the sensations of your breathing. Do this as often as necessary without any form of judgment of yourself.

To experience what it is like to perceive the world with reduced self-identification, try this exercise:

1. Sit down and view your surroundings, taking your time to take everything in.

2. When you are ready, close your eyes and allow yourself to relax.

3. Imagine that you are an alien from a distant planet who has arrived on Earth to study it. You have no information about this world, nor do you have any past experience to draw from. Because of this, you are unable to define, identify, analyze, or judge anything that you experience. In other words, you are a blank slate.

4. Now open your eyes and look at your surroundings again. Take your time.

5. How did your experience observing compare to your first observation?

If you did not notice any difference between the two observations, practice this exercise until you do. Anytime we incorporate our thoughts or judgments while observing, that which is being observed is no longer being viewed in purely as our conceptual thinking is projected onto it. To be able to observe without utilizing conceptual thinking is part of being mindful and present.

The last exercise was a guide to get you to experience seeing without conceptualizing, which is one way to move toward self-love. Anytime we conceptualize our experience, we limit our sense of experience. When we limit our sense of experience, we limit our sense of self due to the self-identification we have developed with our experience.

In the next exercise, you will allow yourself to experience your body through its natural wisdom. You will do this by giving up all resistance toward it by allowing yourself to experience your body and allowing it to express its natural inclinations moment by moment.

Resistance in the Body Meditation

Most instructions for meditation advise you to sit in a comfortable position while seated in an upright position. One of the keys to meditation is learning to allow all experiences and not to control anything. The same happens with the body. In this meditation, you will listen to the body and enable it to move or position itself in complete freedom.

1. Sit down and make yourself comfortable. Allow yourself to relax.

2. Close your eyes and focus on your breath. Allow yourself to become relaxed.

3. Forget about what you learned from your mother about sitting straight. If your body feels like slumping over, let it. Allow your body to do whatever it wants.

4. Place your awareness on the body and its sensations. Let your awareness be soft and do not get caught up in your thinking. Just observe the sensations of the body and any messages that you are getting from the body.

5. Allow yourself to listen to your body for as long as you desire.

Meditations to Increase the Awareness and Allowing of the Body

Now that you have enabled yourself to experience the body without resisting it, you are now ready to increase your awareness of the sensations of the body. For many of us, there is a lack of awareness to our inner world. This is because we spent most of our waking hours focusing on the world outside of ourselves. For the same reason, we often lack an awareness of our bodies. We may be unaware of the subtle sensations and feelings that inhabit it. The body allows our unmanifested self to experience the manifested world.

The sensations of the body, both pleasure and pain, inform us of whether we are in alignment with the highest aspect of ourselves.

1. Sit down, make yourself comfortable, and relax.

2. Close your eyes and allow yourself to follow your breathing during inhalation and exhalation. Place your attention on your breath. Feel it as it courses through your body.

3. Now put your attention on the sensations of the body. Pay attention to any sensation of the body that appears in your awareness.

4. Do you feel a tingling in your hands or feet? Do you feel any tension in your back, shoulders, or face? Do you feel the weight of your body or the pressure on your buttocks from the chair or ground that you are sitting on?

5. Allow yourself to experience the sensations of the body without any judgment of any of them, even the ones that may feel unpleasant. Sensations are just that, sensations. There are no good or bad sensations. Good and bad, pleasant and unpleasant, these are value judgments that exist solely in the mind. The same thing

happens with perceptions, sounds, and thoughts. They just are.

6. Are the sensations that you experience stable? Are they always the same, or do they change? Are they always there, or do they come and go?

7. Just stay in the awareness of your body's sensations. Allow yourself to experience them for as long as you desire.

8. Feel free to allow yourself to continue to meditate on the body for as long as you wish.

What prevents most of us from experiencing a real sense of our power and inner peace is our tendencies to resist, deny, or suppress those emotions and feelings that we find unpleasant. When we do so, we are turning our backs on what is equivalent to our GPS, our navigating system.

Our emotions and feelings are like a compass that informs us of the nature of our thoughts and decision-making. They indicate whether what we are thinking or doing is aligned with our highest good.

When we can allow ourselves to experience our emotions and feelings fully, we can learn to trust ourselves.

Now that you have developed greater awareness to the sensations of your body, you will not apply this awareness to the process of seeing, or more specifically, how you direct your attention.

The Nature of Seeing: Exercise 1

The purpose of this exercise is to experience seeing in a new way:

1. I want you to look at an object in your environment.

2. As you observe this object, notice your attention or awareness. Are you directing your attention or awareness toward the object? If not, bring your awareness or attention toward the object.

3. Rate the quality of your experience on a scale from 1-10.

4. Now, instead of bringing your awareness or attention toward the object, allow the object to come into your awareness. Keep your awareness soft.

5. Now rate your experience. Were you able to detect a difference in your experience? Did you experience a change in the sensations of your body? As with the previous meditations, continue to practice until you can detect a difference.

If you did not notice any differences, please continue to practice the last two meditations until you can perceive a difference or change in your experience of observing.

Please do not attempt the next meditation until you have done so.

The previous meditations mainly focused on how you experience your outer world. In the remaining exercises in this chapter, you will learn how to expand your awareness of your inner world.

Observing Emotions

In this first meditation, you will learn to bring greater awareness to your feelings.

1. Sit down in a comfortable position and close your eyes.

2. Allow yourself to follow your breathing during inhalation and exhalation. Place your attention on your breath. Feel it as it courses through your body.

3. Take on an attitude of complete allowing, that you will have complete acceptance of whatever arises in this meditation.

4. Observe the perceptions, thoughts, sensations, feelings, and emotions that arise within you. Allow them to come and go on their own accord. All you need to do is observe them.

5. Now pay attention to any emotions that arise. Become an observer of them. What happens when your focus is placed on your emotions?

6. Do not give any meaning to the emotions you experience. Do not think of them as being positive or negative. Words such as "positive," "negative," "pleasant," or "unpleasant" are products of the mind.

7. There is no intrinsic meaning to anything in life. All meaning is derived from our minds. Emotions and feelings have no power of their own; they derive all their power from the attention we give them.

8. When observing emotions, do so with complete allowing. Do not try to change anything about them.

9. As you observe your emotions, do you notice a shift in how you experience them? Do they change in intensity? Do they become stronger or milder? Can you locate where the emotions come from? Can you observe where they go?

10. As you observe them, ask yourself "Am I my emotions, or am I the one that is aware of them?" If a feeling or emotion is experienced as being unpleasant, does awareness feel unpleasant? If an emotion is experienced as being pleasant, does awareness feel pleasant?

11. Awareness does not experience anything; it can only know of experience. Awareness is like a beam of light shining on a snow-covered field. The light does not feel

the cold of the snow; it only illuminates it. As you observe emotions, be as the beam of light.

12. This is the end of this meditation. Feel free to remain in meditation for as long as you wish.

The Space Between Thoughts

Now that you have learned to observe your emotions, you will now focus on observing your thoughts. While observing your thoughts is part of the process, the intention of this meditation is to experience the quiet space between your thoughts, which is a step beyond the stillness that you encountered in the exercise at the beginning of Chapter 1.

1. Find a quiet place to sit that is comfortable. You may sit on the floor or in a chair.

2. Close your eyes and allow yourself to relax by placing your attention on the flow of your breathing. Keep your awareness on your breath as you inhale by focusing on the sensations of your breathing. Do the same thing during exhalation by experiencing the sensations as your breath travels out of your body.

3. Breathe naturally. It is important that you make no effort at any time during this meditation.

4. An alternative to following your breathing is to observe the rising and falling of your abdomen.

5. As you breathe, you will experience thoughts, perceptions, sensations, and sounds, and they will have different qualities to them. Some will be pleasant, while others may be uncomfortable or even frightening. Regardless of what you experience, do not interfere with them. Do not try to control, change, or analyze them. Become a scientist who is committed to observing them.

6. Notice how all that you experience is transitory and impermanent. Your thoughts, perceptions, and sensations will appear and then dissolve away.

7. Notice that you are aware of all these mental functions. However, they are not you. You are not your thoughts, perceptions, or sensations.

8. Place your awareness on a thought that you are experiencing. Observe it without judgment or trying to control it. Observe the thought until it fades away. Can you detect where it went?

9. Now place your attention on a thought that is appearing in your awareness. Can you identify where it came from?

10. Now track a thought with your awareness until it fades away. Before the next thought arises, what do you experience?

The space between your thoughts may seem black and empty. Place your attention on this space. As you practice this meditation, you will be able to increase the time you spend in this space. This space indicates that you have transcended the conceptual mind and moved beyond thought. This is the space from which all mental phenomena arise from. With practice, you can access this space anytime you wish. This is your portal to your Buddha nature.

You have completed many meditations to challenge the way that you experience the world around you, as well as the world within you. In the next exercise, you will be challenged to see through the illusions of an "inner" and "outer" world. You will have met the intent of this meditation if you are unable to distinguish between these two worlds.

The Nature of Experiencing:

The following meditation will challenge your beliefs of any separation between your inner and outer world.

Important note: In this meditation, you will be asked a series of questions. When you answer these questions, do not rely on your knowledge, memory, or experience. Respond to these questions based on your immediate and direct experience. Take your time to think before answering. Respond to the questions based on what you experience in the present moment.

1. Sit down and make yourself comfortable and allow yourself to relax. If you would like, you may close your eyes for now.

2. Allow yourself to relax as you focus on your breath. Place your attention on your breath as it enters your body, travels through your body, and then leaves it as you exhale.

3. Breathe normally without exerting any effort. Relax.

4. When you are ready, open your eyes.

5. Now, look at an object in your surroundings.

6. Ask yourself, "Does seeing require any thought or effort?"

7. I am sure you will agree that seeing does not take any effort.

8. As you look at the object, ask yourself "Does seeing stop at the point where the object begins, or do the object and seeing flow into each other?"

9. My hope is that you will agree that seeing and the object being seen flow into each other.

10. Now ask yourself, "Can seeing be known by anything other than seeing?" In other words, how do you know that you are seeing? Can you touch seeing? Can you hear or taste seeing? What is it that knows seeing is taking place?

   That which knows seeing is taking place is awareness, or consciousness. Seeing can only be known. You know that you are seeing because you have an awareness of seeing. Seeing can only be known by the awareness of seeing, and this requires no participation or effort by us.

11. Now ask yourself, "Can the process of seeing be separate from the awareness of seeing?

   I hope that you conclude that seeing and the awareness of seeing are inseparable, just like seeing and the object being seen are inseparable.

12. As you look at the object, ask yourself, "Does seeing occur outside of me or from within me?"

   My hope is that you agree that seeing occurs from within you. Even a blind person, who can "see" mental images, knows this.

13. Now ask yourself, "Is the object that I am viewing within me or outside of me?"

My hope is that you conclude that everything you experience arises from within you, though this is not accurate since "within me" and "outside of me" are just mental concepts. In truth, everything is one.

14. Now reach out and touch your leg. As you touch your leg, ask yourself "Am I experiencing my leg, or am I experiencing the sensation of touching my leg?

    I hope that you agree that you are experiencing the sensation of touching your leg.

15. Now ask yourself, is sensation experienced outside of me or within me?

    I hope you agree that sensation is experienced within you, just like seeing.

16. Now ask yourself, "How do I know sensation is being experienced?"

    You may say, "I know sensation is being experienced because I feel it." This is true, however, how do you know that feeling is being experienced? You know of sensation and feeling because there is awareness of it.

17. Now listen to a sound in your environment. As you listen, ask yourself "Does listening occur outside of me or from within?"

I hope you agree that listening occurs from within you.

18. Now ask yourself, "Are listening and the sound that is heard separate, or do they flow into each other?"

I hope you agree that listening and sound flow into each other.

19. Now ask yourself, "How is listening known?"

Just as with seeing or feeling, listening can only be known through the awareness of it.

I hope you have arrived at the realization that everything we experienced in life is experienced from within and that there is no separation between the awareness of experience and the experience itself. Further, we can never know experience; we can only know of experience. That which is being experienced can never be directly known. This is a most profound and important realization when it applies to self-image, the image we have of ourselves.

You have completed many meditations to challenge how you perceive your experience of your inner and outer worlds. In the last meditation, you challenged the illusion that your inner and outer world are separate from each other. The next and final meditation is the most profound. Though it may seem simple and like a repeat of the last meditations, there is one significant difference. This meditation will cause you to challenge all of your beliefs that you have of who you are.

1. Find a quiet place to sit that is comfortable. You may sit on the floor or in a chair.

2. Close your eyes and allow yourself to relax by placing your attention on the flow of your breath. Keep your awareness on your breath as you inhale by focusing on the sensations of your breathing during inhalation. Place your awareness on your exhalation by focusing on the sensations that you experience as your breath travels out of your body. Breathe naturally; it is important that you make no effort at any time during this meditation. An alternative to following your breath is to observe the rising and falling of your abdomen.

3. As you breathe, you will experience thoughts, perceptions, and sensations, and they will have different qualities to them. Some will be pleasant while others may be uncomfortable or even frightening. Regardless of what you experience, do not interfere with them. Do not try to control, change, or analyze them. Become a scientist who is committed to observing them.

4. As you observe them, be aware that you are the one that is observing these mental functions. You are the one that is observing thought, sensation, and perception. Thus, you cannot be these things. Try to find the one that is doing the observing. Keep in mind that anything that you can detect with your awareness cannot be the one that is doing the observing, for it is also observed.

How was your experience with the last meditation? Was it frustrating? Did you feel that you could not do it? Were you unable to find that which you refer to as "I"? If this was your experience, do not be disappointed. You made the most profound realization that you could have. The reason why you were unable to find the "I" that was observing the coming and going of thoughts, sensations, and perceptions is that it does not exist! What you refer to as "I" is just another thought which is being observed by the larger consciousness. As I stated before, the greater consciousness cannot be perceived or experienced. But it is the knower of all experiences.

My hope is that you will come to realize that your experience of having weight issues is just a thought that has been attracted by the thought of "I," which you have personalized. In truth, both of these thoughts ("weight issues" and "I") are just two of the innumerable thoughts that are witnessed by your higher self, that eternal aspect of you that remains untouched by experience.

By doing these exercises, you will lessen your sense of self-identification with the phenomenal world (that which can be perceived, including thoughts, sensations, and perceptions). Additionally, you will expand your ability to become a conscious manifester and become happier and healthier, which is the subject of the next section.

Group 3

The purpose of the previous exercises was to increase your sense of awareness of your "inner world" while at the same time reducing your sense of identification with your mind and body. Hopefully, these exercises have led you to a direct experience of yourself that is beyond the illusions of the mind and body. If you had difficulty with these activities, please continue to practice them until you have the direct experience that who you are is beyond the mind and body.

Though I ask you to practice these exercises, it is important that you do not do them just for the sake of doing them. Each time you practice them, you want to practice them as though you were doing them for the first time. Also, when doing the exercises, do not "try" to do them. There should be no effort on your part other than getting yourself to do them. It is not the purpose of doing these exercises to do them continually until you "get them right." Rather, it is about an exploration of the ever-expanding dimensions of consciousness.

If you feel comfortable with the past exercises, it is time to advance to the next step of the process, which is applying the Law of Attraction to weight loss. Before doing these exercises, I am going to ask you to go on a diet for one day to prepare yourself. You may be thinking "What? I thought this book was about not dieting!" If this is what you are saying to yourself, you are correct. However, the diet I am referring to is the "resistance diet."

The One-Day Resistance Diet

One of the reasons I offered you the previous exercises was because they all involved letting go of any resistance you may have been experiencing within your life. To give up resistance to our thoughts, sensations, and perceptions is a huge step toward loving ourselves and employing the Law of Attraction effectively. This exercise takes the releasing of resistance to a whole new level, the releasing of resistance toward daily living.

I want you to spend one day where you do not engage in any activity that you feel resistant to. If it does not feel right to you, do not do it. Only engage in those activities that resonate with you, that you feel good about doing. If you find yourself having trouble doing this exercise, start off small by telling yourself you will not do anything for the next hour that you feel resistant to and then gradually increase the time until you can do it for a whole day.

Most people will have difficulty with this exercise, and some will point out that this exercise is unrealistic. We all have to do certain things, and whether we like it or not, there is no choice. These types of sentiments are the sole property of our conditioned minds as well as our sense of identification as a person rather than our higher nature. I realize that as long as we live in this dimension that we call "daily life," there will be things that we need to take care of. To address these situations, here are some simple guidelines:

Change your perspective of the task that is creating resistance in you by focusing on all the benefits that you would gain by completing it.

Find ways to change the way that you approach doing the task by making it more enjoyable for yourself. For example: Listen to your favorite music while cleaning the house, or invite a friend over to do your taxes together.

If none of the previous techniques work, do not take on the task until you have come to accept the fact that you need to do this task and that it will not be enjoyable. Regarding this technique, I want you to focus on the word "accept." It means that you do the task with complete acceptance for what it is. You have lost any sense of putting up a fight against it.

Hopefully, you have come to the insight that the activities in our lives have nothing to with the level of resistance that we experience in our lives. Rather, it is us projecting our sense of resistance onto the activity.

Trusting our Decisions

The previous exercises provided you with an opportunity to develop greater self-awareness, become more in tune with your mind and body, and lower your resistance. All of these things lead to the development of trust in our lives. Trust is crucial in successfully employing the Law of Attraction and losing weight because there are so many competing forces to distract us or create doubt in our minds.

We often think of wisdom as arising from our mind or brain. However, this is inaccurate. I ask you to consider that the body has a wisdom of its own, a wisdom that is superior to the rational mind.

The mind can only understand concepts, that which cannot be observed, measured, weighed, touched, or heard does not register with the mind.

The body's wisdom can understand information that is beyond the phenomenal world. The last few meditations were intended to increase your awareness of the body. You will now use that awareness to tap into the wisdom of the body.

1. Sit down in a comfortable position and close your eyes.

2. Allow yourself to follow your breath during inhalation and exhalation. Place your attention on your breathing. Feel it as it courses through your body. Allow yourself to relax.

3. I want you to think of a decision that you need to make. If you currently do not have a decision to make, create one that is relevant to you.

4. Now that you have a decision to make, think of the different choices that are available to you when making your decision.

5. Now think of the potential consequences for each choice, if you selected it. For example, if I had to make a decision on whether to buy a new car, I would consider the potential consequence for each choice I am considering. If I decide to buy the car, the consequence could be that I have a new car, but I will have no more savings.

    When doing this part of the meditation, do not overanalyze the situation. Just go with whatever answer comes to you. This is not intended to be an intellectual meditation.

6. Now return your attention to your breath and allow yourself to relax. Do not engage with any of your

thoughts, allow yourself to relax and become still within.

7. Now, while remaining in your peacefulness, I want you to review your potential choices, one by one. Consider each choice separately, giving it your full attention.

8. As you review the choice, ask yourself "Should I say yes to this decision?" When you do this, pay attention to the sensations of the body. Observe the sensations of the body.

9. When you think of this choice, do you feel constricted or relaxed? Is your breathing relaxed or shallow? Does your chest feel hard or soft? Does your body feel stiff or tingly? Notice the sensations of the body and the quality of your breathing as you reflect on each option.

10. Without exception, you were intended to be happy in this life. Happiness is your birthright. Which option brings your body the greatest sense of peacefulness? Which option brings about the greatest ease in your breathing? Regardless of what your mind or conventional wisdom says, that is the option that is right for you.

Transforming Feelings

Earlier in this book, it was indicated that our feelings are like a GPS in that they indicate our alignment with the universe.

Hopefully, you also have come to the realization that any sense of separation between your inner and outer world are illusionary. Further, I have indicated that everything arises from consciousness. Having said of all this, I will now offer you some little-known insight, which is this: There is nothing in this world that can make you feel anything. Rather, you project your feelings on your experiences.

While our feelings are our GPS regarding our alignment, our feelings are constantly changing, as is everything else in the phenomenal world. While feelings indicate our alignment, the feelings themselves are transitory. When we have a change in feelings regarding anything in life, that change has nothing to do with the object or feelings themselves. Our feelings change due to us changing our focus. In other words, how we focus on anything in life determines whether we are aligned with our higher selves. Everything else is irrelevant. These understandings point to one grand truth: You are the creator of all meaning and the witness to all of experience. Everything you experience is a projection of yourself! The next two meditations will guide you in transforming your feelings.

Exercise 1

1. Sit down, close your eyes, and relax.

2. Allow yourself to become silent and observe the thoughts, feeling, emotions, and sensations that arise

within. Allow all of these phenomena to present themselves to your awareness.

3. Relax.

4. I want you to think of a situation that is currently causing you feelings of uneasiness, concern, or hurt. When you identify such a situation, allow yourself to focus on it. Relive the experience in your mind.

5. As you focus on the situation, become aware of the feelings that arise. Allow the feelings to arise naturally. Remember, your feelings are like a compass, they have a message for you. They are telling you to move toward or away from that which you are focusing on. When we are making decisions, taking actions, or focusing on things that bring about pleasant feelings, we know that we are on the right track by being consistent with our sense of integrity. Conversely, when we have feelings that are unpleasant, we are experiencing situations that are inconsistent with our sense of integrity.

6. Now ask yourself, "What can I do, believe, or focus on that will make me feel better about this situation?" Is there a decision that you need to make? Do you need to let go of something? Do you need to question your thinking? Do you need to take time for yourself? Do you need to risk disappointing others?

7. Keep inquiring with yourself until you have identified a way to address the situation that leaves you with feelings of relief, calm, or peace.

8. If the answer you come up with to deal with the situation leads to positive feelings, trust that this is the correct decision for you. Your feelings are completely accurate and reliable for you at this moment of time. If your feelings regarding your solution or the situation change, honor them as well.

9. Be sure not to confuse your feelings for your thoughts or beliefs. Your feelings are reliable; however, your thoughts and beliefs are not.

10. If you are unable to find a way to make yourself feel better, that is okay also. Allow yourself to remain with the feeling. Offer your full acceptance to this feeling. Accepting our feelings and being at peace with them is an act of self- love and an indication of integrity.

Exercise 2

1. Sit in a comfortable position and close your eyes.

2. Allow yourself to follow your breathing during inhalation and exhalation. Place your attention on your breath. Feel it as it courses through your body.

3. Just as we did in the previous meditation, I want to think about a situation that concerns you. As you think of this situation, observe the emotions and feelings that arise from within you. Be aware of the sensations of your body and your ability to breathe freely.

4. Now ask yourself, "Why does this situation bother me? What does this situation mean to me?" As you answer these questions, pay attention to the feelings, sensations, and emotions that you are experiencing.

5. Now ask yourself, "That which I am experiencing, what does it feel like?" For example, you may be experiencing tension or anxiety. Using this example, the next question you would ask yourself would be, "What does tension or anxiety feel like?" Perhaps for you, anxiety makes your body feel constricted or heavy.

6. Notice that the question was not what you think about tension or anxiety. Do not involve your thoughts in this process. Ask yourself, "What does it FEEL like?" Allow yourself to get in touch with what your experience feels like.

7. Do not worry about the words you use, focus on identifying the feeling. Make sure that you continue to breathe as you experience the feeling. Allow yourself to dive into the feeling.

8. Whatever your response was to the last question, ask yourself "What does this feel like?" Going back to the previous example, if anxiety feels like your body is constricted and heavy, you would then ask, "What does being constricted and heavy feel like?" Whatever answer comes to you, you would then observe that experience, making sure that you continue to breathe as you allow yourself to fully experience the feelings.

9. Whatever your response was to the last question, ask yourself, "What does this feel like?" If my response was that being constricted and heavy feels like I am being crushed by a boulder, I would ask myself, "What does it feel like being crushed by a boulder?"

   This is the format for this meditation, continuously asking yourself, "What does it feel like?" and then diving into the feeling or emotion, allowing yourself to fully experience it, all the time breathing normally.

10. When you continuously ask these questions and allow yourself to fully experience the feelings that are associated with the emotion, the emotion will transform on its own.

11. You will know when you have reached the end when the emotion that was previously unpleasant begins to feel pleasant or neutral.

12. You can also use this same meditation on positive emotions, in which case the positive feeling of the emotion will expand.

13. Repeat this meditation until you can successfully transform a negative emotion. Just for clarification, emotions are not positive or negative. They feel negative or positive by the meaning that we give them. This is why this meditation works. You are changing the meaning that you give an emotion by placing your attention on it.

Healing Your Relationships with Others

Because there is no separation between our inner and outer worlds, the outer world is a mirror of our inner world. All problems in relationships are due to us projecting the qualities of our inner world onto the other person. The following is a meditation to transforming your inner world, which will transform that which you are projecting on the other person.

In this meditation, you will reduce the power of a belief by using self-inquiry. Most of us do not question our beliefs, we assume them to be true.

As mentioned before, beliefs are thoughts that we have devoted a lot of our attention to. They have become very powerful because of the attention they have received from us, and they become ingrained in us. We frequently act on these beliefs without even being aware of the belief itself.

The following meditation is based on our relationships with others. However, this meditation can be applied to any situation.

1. Sit down in a comfortable position and close your eyes.

2. Allow yourself to follow your breath during inhalation and exhalation. Place your attention on your breath. Feel it as it courses through your body.

3. I want you to think of someone who you believe treated you in an unfair or unjust way. It can be recently or in the past. When you have this person in mind, I want you to relieve the specific situation where this person mistreated you.

4. Where did the situation take place?

5. Imagine the surroundings of this location.

6. Where was this person when the situation happened? What were they doing at the time? See it in your mind; visualize it in as much detail as possible.

7. Where were you at the time? What were you doing when the situation happened?

8. What did they say or do to you that caused you to become angry or hurt?

9. How did you feel when the situation happened? What did it feel like? What did you tell yourself?

10. Remember the meditation earlier in this program where you were challenged to observe the nature of seeing?

   You were asked to determine if the object you were viewing was outside of you or within you. As you relive the situation where this person hurt you, determine if this situation is within you or outside of you.

   Remember, our thoughts and emotions have no power other than what we give them. Why do you continue to give this memory power?

   Can you say that you are absolutely sure that this person intended to hurt you? Our emotions and feelings arise from within us, and so do our perceptions. Did this person really harm you, or are you projecting your thoughts, feelings, and emotions on this person?

11. I want you to replay this situation in your mind a second time. This time, I want you to do something different. I want you to look at this person who you believe hurt you, but discard any thoughts or emotions

that you have for that person. Just observe them without judgment, stay as the observer. What are they doing? Did this person attempt to do anything to you?

12. Now ask yourself this question: "Am I doing that which I believe this person did to me to myself? If this is true, how can I be more loving and forgiving toward myself?"

In case you have not realized it yet, all of our experiences are a reflection of the experiences that we have within ourselves. We can never know anyone, nor is it possible to have a relationship with another person. All we have is our perceptions of the other person. What we call a relationship is a relationship with our perceptions.

Application of the Law of Attraction for Weight Loss

"The greatest revolution of our generation is the discovery that human beings, by changing the inner attitudes of their minds, can change the outer aspects of their lives."
William James

I want to congratulate you for reaching this point in the book. That you have reached this point demonstrates that you are committed to changing your life and losing weight. This is the part of the book where the rubber meets the road. You have learned a lot about your relationship with consciousness and experience, and you have learned about the role of your thoughts, emotions, and feelings. You have also practiced a number of meditations for expanding your awareness. Now it is time to take what you have learned and apply it to weight loss.

Let us start off with a quick review of why we experience weight problems. We experience emotional pains in our life in which we suppress or deny our feelings. The suppression or denial of these emotional pains results in them either being blocked by our subconscious, or we distract ourselves to avoid dealing with them. Either way, these emotional aspects of ourselves attract conditions that are of the same energetic level into our lives. We overeat as a way of comforting ourselves from our experience of life.

We want to raise our energy level so that we attract the conditions that we desire. To raise our energy level and experience the higher-level emotions, we need to uncover the root beliefs that we are holding and replace them with beliefs that empower us. We also want to lower our resistance to our experiences so that it does not compete with our intentions for what we want in our life.

There is an easy way to remember all of this:

We want to:

- Open ourselves to experiencing all of our thoughts, emotions, and feelings without any judgment.
- After accepting our disempowering thoughts, emotions, and feelings, we want to transform them into more empowering ones.
- Honor ourselves by not engaging in any behaviors or activities that cause us to experience resistance.
- Remember that the quality of our experiences reflects the quality of our inner world. When we transform our inner world, we transform our experience of our outer world, including our physical body.

There are exercises in this book for addressing each one of these points. The following is a case study to illustrate how this works.

Mary has struggled with her weight all of her life. Since she was a child, she tried to please her parents, but nothing she ever did seemed to appease them. Nothing ever seemed to be good enough for them. To gain some sense of control in her life, Mary started using food. Any time she felt a sense of uncertainty, Mary reached for food. Though the food comforted her, it resulted in her packing on the pounds. Her increasing weight added to her feelings of insecurity, which she would numb by reaching for food.

Though Mary tried to diet and lose weight a number of times in her adult life, she was never successful. She would either be thrown off her diet whenever she experienced stress so she would not lose weight, or she would lose weight, but regained it due to her returning to eating when a stressor entered her life.

Like most of us, Mary's sense of identity came from her body and mind. She based her sense of identity on what she saw in the mirror or in the way others looked at her. Her sense of identity was affected by the media, which serves a 24-hour cocktail of glamorous people and diet products.

Mary has learned to suppress her painful emotions while compensating for her insecurity by giving the impression that she is in control of her life. At work, she is an overachiever and takes on every project that she can sign up for, and she has positioned herself to be the "go-to" person.

While she is a star performer at work, she finds her work exhausting. In her private life, she finds herself involved with a lot of drama with her family and friends by getting involved with other peoples' business. By living this way, she distracts herself from experiencing the feelings that she is inadequate as a person. Mary's professional and personal life is no accident; she attracted them into her life through the Law of Attraction. Remember, Mary suppressed her feelings that nothing that she ever did for her parents was good enough. Although these feelings are suppressed, they still attract the conditions that are an energetic match. Because she is unaware of these feelings, they trump any conscious intent that she may have for her life, such as losing weight. She is unable to lose weight because she is continuously being triggered by her environment, and her conditioned response has been to reach for food.

Now, let us imagine that Mary decides to follow what she learned in this book and follows the exercises as outlined. She not only does these exercises, but she practices them until she is comfortable with them. By doing the belief exercises in

Group 1, Mary would discover the root belief that she has suppressed. Her root belief no longer has the potency that it had when it was suppressed. By bringing her root belief into her field of awareness, it is automatically diminished in its power to attract those conditions that are causing her suffering.

By adopting a new empowering belief, Mary has shifted her focus in the direction of that which she desires for her life. By taking daily actions that are consistent with her new empowering belief, that belief is gaining power from the attention that she is giving it. Because this belief is becoming more powerful, its ability to attract that which she desires will also gain strength. Mary's increased attention on her new beliefs means the energy she exerted to suppress her old beliefs will be freed up. The freeing up of energy means that her resistance toward her suppressed beliefs has been released.

Doing any of the meditation exercises brings her even further in the transformation process because it allows her to develop the realization that she was never her thoughts, sensations, or perceptions. Rather, she is the awareness that is observing these mental phenomena. Because she realizes that she is the observer, she has gone from personally identifying with her mental phenomena to developing space between her and that which she is witnessing. Because she has developed this space, her reactivity to their presence has diminished. She realizes that these mental phenomena are powerless without her attention. Another benefit of meditation is that the sense of separation she has with the world around her has dissolved as her sense of connection with all she experiences deepens.

By doing the exercises in Group 3, Mary learned how to pay attention to her feelings and not doing anything that she feels resistant to. By listening to her feelings, she has learned to trust them. Because she has learned to trust her feelings, she makes better decisions. She has also learned to transform her feelings anytime that she experiences feeling that make her feel disempowered. By doing the last meditation, Healing Your Relationships with Others, Mary has changed her past by changing the way she experiences it.

Every dynamic that has created suffering in her has collapsed. Mary has learned self-love and that self-love puts her in perfect alignment to attract into her life that which she desires.

Creating a 30-Day Plan

I have titled this section *Creating a 30-Day Plan*; however, you can increase or decrease this time period so that it best fits your needs. Everyone is at a different place in their spiritual development. Further, the exercises in this book are for you to practice continuously, not only to develop competency, but also to raise and maintain your life condition. In this section, I have outlined key points for how to implement these exercises into your daily life. Once you develop as sense of comfort and familiarity with the exercises, you can make adjustments to personalize your own plan. Until then, I recommend you follow this outline:

Day 1:

From Group 1, do the *Ultimate Why* and one of the exercises under *Turning the Tables on a Root Belief*. It is important that you follow the exercises exactly as described. Also, unless you are already familiar with meditation, I encourage you to do the first exercise. It is also important that you review the results of this exercise daily until you internalize it, meaning that you experience the emotional pain of continuing with your current belief and excitement for your new empowering belief.

Though this exercise is scheduled for Day 1, use the exercises in Group 1 anytime you experience yourself holding on to a disempowering belief. Though you may remove the root cause belief, other disempowering beliefs can take its place until you have developed a higher life condition.

Day 2:

Unless you are already experienced in meditation, do the *Basic Meditation* in Group 2. Though this is a simple meditation, it will provide you with a foundation for the more advanced meditations that follow. Continue to practice this meditation until you feel comfortable with it. Do not proceed with the more advanced meditations until you have this one under your belt. Even if you find yourself having to practice this mediation for a solid month, it will be well worth it. It will provide you with numerous benefits and insights to help you achieve your desires for weight loss.

The second and third exercises in this group can be practiced at any time since you do not need to develop your meditation skills. I recommend you do these exercises as often as you like, but I want you to do them at least once. They are invaluable in creating greater awareness to the act of perception and the experiencing of resistance in the body.

Days 3-8

Practice the remaining meditations in Group 2 in the order that they are sequenced. You can practice one meditation per day. After you have tried out these meditations, decide which ones resonate with you the most and practice them every day for the remaining 22 days.

Day 9

From Group 3, do the *One-Day Resistant Diet*. I encourage you to repeat this exercise whenever you want. The more that you do this exercise, the more you will recondition yourself for success in weight loss or anything else that you desire.

Day 10

From Group 3, do *Trusting Our Decisions*. Practice this exercise as often you can for the remaining 20 days. If you can become skillful in this exercise, you will have an exercise that will serve you for life!

Days 11-13

Practice the remaining meditations in Group 3 in the order that they are sequenced. Practice one meditation per day. After you have tried out these meditations, decide which ones resonate with you the most and practice them every day for the remaining 17 days.

Days 14-30

Practice the exercises from Groups 2 and 3 that you have selected, plus, the following exercises as needed: Group 1 (All of them); Group 2: *Basic Meditation, Resistance in the Body Meditation,* and any of the meditations to increase the awareness and allowing of the body. Group 3: *Trusting Our Decisions.*

By giving all of these exercises a sincere attempt and practicing those exercises that feel right to you, you will develop a shift in consciousness where you will start perceiving yourself and the world around you differently. Rather than focusing on your flaws or your relationship with others, you will start experiencing an inner knowing of your truth that is bathed in a greater sense of calm and equanimity.

Intention and Meditation

There is a reason why the majority of the exercises in this book involve meditation. The practice of meditation is the single most important skill that you can develop to effectively use the Law of Attraction. It is common, especially in Western societies, to associate the practice of meditation with stress relief or for calming the mind. While meditation does address these things, the practice of meditation is so much more. The practice of meditation allows us to challenge the way we perceive ourselves and our relationship to life. By allowing ourselves to take on the role of an observer rather than the role of the one who is engaged with their thoughts, we have the opportunity to achieve an amazing realization: There is no separation between the knowing of experience and experience itself. You were presented with an opportunity to experience this through the exercises in this book, especially in the Group 2 Exercise, *The Nature of Experiencing*.

I will leave you with two important points to follow as your practice the Law of Attraction through the use of meditation. Given that there is no separation between you and the universe, all you need to do to attract weight loss is offer a clear signal to the universe of your intentions. Your intentions are what are communicated to the universe, and your intentions will determine how the universe responds back. Here are some points to consider when creating your attentions:

State your intentions in the positive

If your intentions are to lose weight, you will more likely attract what you want if your intentions are, "I want to be happier and healthier" than if your intentions are, "I want to lose 30 pounds." There are two reasons for this. The first reason is that when you have the intention, "I want to lose 30 pounds," you are focusing on your weight. When you focus on your weight, you may experience disempowering emotions. More importantly, you are expressing resistance to an aspect of yourself. Further, "I want to lose 30 pounds" is a very specific intention, which limits how the universe can respond back. To better understand this, I will use the example of an artist who is commissioned by a client to create an inspiring painting for them. Which request do you think will yield the best results from the artist?

A) The client tells the artist to paint an inspiring painting.
B) The client tells the artist to paint an inspiring painting and then goes on to tell the artist what colors he needs to use, the kind of brush he needs to use, and the exact dimensions of the painting.

Obviously, the first option is going to provide the artist with more freedom to express his or her creativity and achieve the outcomes that the client is expecting than the second option. This is why the intention, "I want to be happier and healthier," is a more powerful intention. It places your focus on what you want; it provides greater possibilities for creative expression by the universe, and it does not provide room for resistance to express itself.

Employ your emotions

The second point I want to share with you is the power of emotions. There is a widespread misunderstanding that the Law of Attraction is activated by our thoughts, and that we attract what we think. While this is true, it is only a partial truth. Our emotions are a superior force for manifesting in our life, which is why you were provided with a number of exercises involving emotions. Rather than just releasing your intentions during meditation, generate the emotions that you would experience if your intentions were already realized in your life.

From the perspective of higher levels of consciousness, it is impossible to separate that which you desire from yourself! The only thing that separates you from that which you desire is the perspective that you are a separate and distinct being who lives in a physical world. From the perspective of higher consciousness, you are like a drop in the ocean or a breeze traveling through the air. Any difficulty in weight loss is due to this sense of separation. The exercises in this book, if practiced with an open heart and open mind, will enable you to come to this realization. When this is understood, you will not have to try to lose weight, it will happen on its own. It will happen on its own because you will be living your life aligned with the highest aspect of yourself.

This book is also available in audio format.

You can learn more at:

www.LOAforSuccess.com/audiobooks

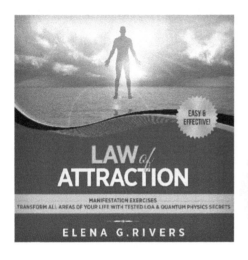 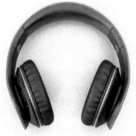

Conclusion

We are approaching the end of this book now. Remember that the Law of Attraction is not an end unto itself. It is just a normal function of the universe and we can learn to use it consciously. However, the greatest things happen after diving deep and developing more awareness.

Upon achieving higher levels of awareness, it will become crystal clear to you that who we are is beyond our thoughts. As pure consciousness, we can manifest anything we want spontaneously without bigger effort. In order to get there, get committed to getting to know your true self and removing resistance. Schedule your LOA rituals time and enjoy the exercises from this book. We are all energy. Let's rise higher and enjoy the process! I am very curious to hear back to you.

If you have a few moments, please share your thoughts in the review section of this book and let us know which exercise you found most helpful. Your honest review would be much appreciated. It's you I am writing for and I would love to know your feedback.

Enjoy your LOA journey,

Elena

A Special Offer from Elena

Finally, I would like to invite you to join my private mailing list (my **VIP LOA Newsletter**). Whenever I release a new book, you will be able to get it at a discounted price (or sometimes even for free, but don't tell anyone 😊).

In the meantime, I will keep you entertained with a free copy of my exclusive LOA workbook that will be emailed to you when you sign up.

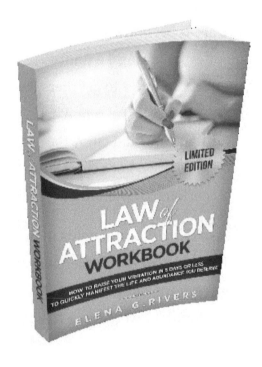

To join visit the link below now:

www.loaforsuccess.com/newsletter

After you have signed up, you will get a free instant access to this exclusive workbook (+ many other helpful resources that I will be sending you on a regular basis). I hope you will enjoy your free workbook.

If you have any questions, please email us at: support@loaforsuccess.com

More Books written by Elena G.Rivers

Available at: www.loaforsuccess.com

Ebook – Paperback – Audiobook Editions Available Now

Law of Attraction for Amazing Relationships

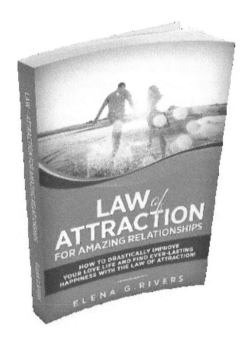

Law of Attraction -Manifestation Exercises

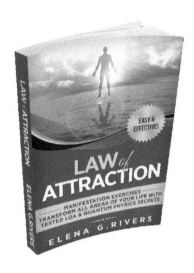

Law of Attraction for Abundance

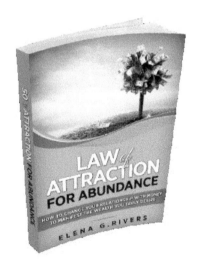

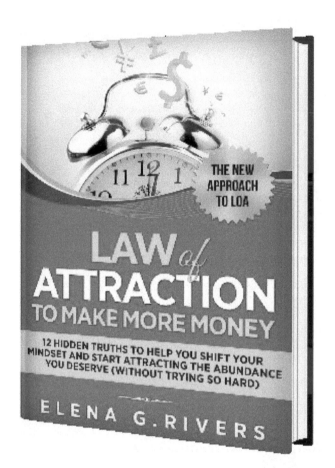

You will find more at:

www.loaforsuccess.com/books

Lightning Source UK Ltd.
Milton Keynes UK
UKHW020644280422
402201UK00009B/640